# ...ISLE

the last date shown below.

# MADELEINE
# LEININGER

# Notes on Nursing Theories

### SERIES EDITORS

Chris Metzger McQuiston
*Doctoral Candidate, Wayne State University*

Adele A. Webb
*College of Nursing, University of Akron*

**Notes on Nursing Theories** is a series of monographs designed to provide the reader with a concise description of conceptual frameworks and theories in nursing. Each monograph includes a biographical sketch of the theorist, origin of the theory, assumptions, concepts, propositions, examples for application to practice and research, a glossary of terms, and a bibliography of classic works, critiques, and research.

# MADELEINE LEININGER

## Cultural Care Diversity and Universality Theory

### Cheryl L. Reynolds
### Madeleine Leininger

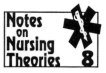

Notes
on
Nursing
Theories   8

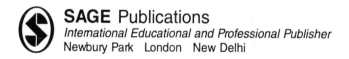

**SAGE** Publications
*International Educational and Professional Publisher*
Newbury Park   London   New Delhi

*For information address:*

SAGE Publications, Inc.
2455 Teller Road
Newbury Park, California 91320

SAGE Publications Ltd.
6 Bonhill Street
London EC2A 4PU
United Kingdom

SAGE Publications India Pvt. Ltd.
M-32 Market
Greater Kailash I
New Delhi 110 048 India

Printed in the United States of America

**Library of Congress Cataloging-in-Publication Data**

Reynolds, Cheryl L.
    Madeleine Leininger: cultural care diversity and universality theory / Cheryl L. Reynolds, Madeleine Leininger.
        p. cm. — (Notes on nursing theories; v. 8)
    Portions of this book are a shorthand version of Leininger's book, *Culture care diversity and universality*, published by the National League for Nursing in 1991.
    Includes bibliographical references.
    ISBN 0-8039-5097-7 (cl). — ISBN 0-8039-5098-5 (pbk.)
    1. Transcultural nursing. 2. Nursing—Cross-cultural studies. 3. Nursing—Social aspects. 4. Health behavior—Cross-cultural studies. 5. Nursing—Philosophy. 6. Leininger, Madeleine M. I. Leininger, Madeleine M. II. Culture care diversity and universality. III. Title. IV. Series.
    [DNLM: 1. Nursing Theory. 2. Transcultural Nursing. WY 101 R462m 1993]
RT86.54.C85 1993
510.73'01—DC20
DNLM/DLC                                       93-5728

    95 96 10 9 8 7 6 5 4 3 2
Sage Production Editor: Diane S. Foster

# Contents

To Mom and Dad,
the first people to teach me the meaning of caring.
—Cheryl

# Series Editors' Foreword

The purpose of this series of monographs is to provide the reader with a concise description of conceptual frameworks and theories in nursing. It is not intended to replace the primary works of nurse theorists, but to provide direction for their use. Designed for the undergraduate student, these monographs will also be helpful guides for graduate students and faculty.

Due to the complexity of existing books and chapters on nursing conceptual frameworks and theories, students often have difficulty understanding and incorporating nursing theory into their practice. The concise monographs of this series include a biosketch of the theorist, origin of the theory, assumptions, concepts, propositions, examples for application to practice and research, glossary of terms, and a bibliography of classic works, critiques, and research. Organization of the information in this manner will facilitate student understanding and use, thereby broadening the base of nursing science.

CHRIS METZGER MCQUISTON
ADELE A. WEBB

# Foreword

In keeping with the purpose of the **Notes on Nursing Theories** series of monographs on nursing theories, this publication has been primarily prepared for undergraduate nursing students and their instructors to provide an overview of basic information about *Culture Care Diversity and Universality: A Theory of Nursing*. Undoubtedly, nursing students as well as interested colleagues will be eager to learn about a theory that is growing in relevance and usefulness worldwide.

In a world that is rapidly becoming multicultural, it is imperative that nurses consider theories that help them to discover relevant dimensions of nursing. It is timely that nursing students study theories that make them think about the care of people from diverse cultures in relation to health, human care, and illness. The theory of culture care focuses on generating knowledge related to the nursing care of people who value their cultural heritage and life ways. The theory has great significance because nurses are realizing that today, and even more in the near future, they need knowledge to guide them in their decisions and actions as they care for clients of different cultures.

As a culture care theorist, I have devoted a lifetime of creative thinking to developing the theory so that it could be used in all cultures to study and discover culture care differences (the diversities) and similarities (the universals) about transcultural human care. Accordingly, the theory with research findings is viewed not only as highly relevant but also as a powerful and meaningful theory to understand human beings of diverse cultures. The theory, and findings from the use of the theory, will remain important well into the 21st century because of increased multiculturalism worldwide.

Currently, nurses are traveling and working in many foreign cultures. However, they often realize, by cultural shock or in other ways, that people differ in the way they view professional nursing and client care needs. Nurses are almost forced to consider the role of cultural factors in client care.

The culture care theory has helped many nurses to focus on the diverse cultural factors that influence client behavior and well being. And since culture is holistic and comprehensive, the nurse discovers important *emic* (local) views and well as *etic* (outsider's) views to develop nursing care practices. Data from the culture care theory will also assist nurses to avoid cultural imposition and other unfavorable nursing care practices. Most important, the theory with concomitant research findings often becomes a "blueprint" to guide nursing decisions, actions, and outcomes for quality-based nursing care practices. The theory also supports the work of transcultural nursing specialists or generalists as they use culture-specific knowledge generated from the theory. The theory and transcultural nursing have been evolving together for 3 decades, bringing many new benefits to nurses and clients.

The authors of this volume have, therefore, brought together an overview of the theory of culture care with a focus on the origin and the development of the theory over time. They have provided highlights of the theory using the well-known sunrise model to depict and study the components of the theory in Western and non-Western cultures. It has always been exciting to see nurses who use the theory greatly expand their thinking as they realize different cultural factors that influence illness, wellness, and ways clients maintain their wellness or become ill. The authors present fundamental perspectives of the theory to help students discover new facts, insights, meanings, and expressions about culture care that can change nursing practices significantly in providing culture-congruent care as the goal of the theory. Students will find the content fascinating and different as they shift from traditional medical model symptoms and disease orientations to cultural ways of knowing.

Chapter 2 of this mini-theory book is actually a shorthand version of Leininger's comprehensive and definitive work about her theory, *Culture Care Diversity and Universality: A Theory of Nursing*, published by the National League for Nursing, 1991. (The reader is, therefore, encouraged to read the 1991 book to gain more in-depth insights about the theory and the ethnonursing research method.) In this volume, there are several research studies and findings of nearly 30 cultures to guide nurses' thinking for Leininger's three models of nursing practice. Some very practical ways to use the research findings from many different cultures are discussed with the transcultural nursing research studies of different cultures.

Finally, one must commend Adele Webb and Chris McQuiston, editors of the series, who were doctoral students in the College of Nursing at Wayne State University when this series was launched. They recognized the need to help undergraduate students and other readers learn about and understand definitive characteristics of nursing theories in as simple and informative a manner as possible. They saw the need to incorporate theoretical ideas early into baccalaureate nursing programs so that theory and clinical practices could be used by students throughout their studies. I, therefore, applaud Adele Webb and Chris McQuiston for their leadership with the **Notes on Nursing Theories** series, and their genuine desire to facilitate student learning about nursing theorists as well as the critical importance of nursing theories to advance nursing knowledge.

MADELEINE M. LEININGER, RN, CTN, PhD, LHD, DS, FAAN
Professor of Nursing and Anthropology
Colleges of Nursing and Liberal Arts,
Wayne State University, Detroit, Michigan

# Biographical Sketch of the Nurse Theorist: Madeleine M. Leininger, PhD, RN, CTN, LHD, FAAN

Born: July 6, 1924, Sutton, Nebraska
Current Position: Professor of Nursing and Anthropology,
　　Wayne State University, Detroit, Michigan
Education: Diploma at St. Anthony's School of Nursing,
　　Denver, Colorado, 1948
BS Biological Science, Benedictine College, Atchison, Kansas,
　　1950
MSN Catholic University of America, Washington, DC, 1954
PhD Anthropology, University of Washington, Seattle,
　　Washington, 1965
Fellow, American Academy of Nursing
Honorary Doctor of Humane Letters, Benedictine College, 1975
Honorary Doctor of Science: University of Indianapolis,
　　Indianapolis, Indiana
Honorary Doctor of Nursing Science: University of Kuopio,
　　Kuopio, Finland (Only woman nurse scientist and
　　anthropologist to receive this degree)
Editor, *Journal of Transcultural Nursing*
Founder, transcultural nursing field and Transcultural Nursing
　　Society
President, International Association of Human Caring
Recipient of numerous awards and honors

# 1

## Origin of Leininger's Theory

CHERYL L. REYNOLDS

Through clinical practice with disturbed children while developing the role of the clinical specialist in child psychiatric nursing, Leininger became aware that cultural differences between patients and nurses made a difference in health outcomes. Children of diverse cultures reacted to the interventions of nurses differently. Thus Leininger credits children with pointing out that culture was the link to understanding the nursing care of persons from different backgrounds. This discovery led her to study cultural differences in the perceptions of care in 1954 and doctoral work in cultural anthropology in 1959 (Leininger, 1980; 1988a).

Leininger was concerned with "ways that care and nursing practice could accurately describe and reflect nursing knowledge" (Leininger, 1988a, p. 152). This search, coupled with the discovery of culture as the missing link in nursing theory, set the stage for Leininger to determine that "care and culture were inextricably linked together and could not be separated in nursing care actions and decisions" (Leininger, 1988a, p. 153).

Doctoral study in anthropology and a background in nursing provided Leininger with expertise in two major disciplines—both of which support the concept of holism and have as their object knowledge of human phenomena (Leininger, 1970). With an understanding of how anthropology could contribute to nursing knowledge and how nursing could contribute to anthropological knowledge, Leininger began to look at the practice and discipline of nursing in a new way.

Leininger became interested in questions about "the role of caring and curing in human evolution and survival of the species" (Leininger, 1980, p. 137). Through observation she determined that medical practice was oriented toward curing while nursing was oriented toward "caring acts and processes focusing on multiple factors influencing wellness and illness" (Leininger, 1980, p. 137). The result of reflecting on this difference was Leininger's conclusion that patterns of human caring and curing could be identified if anthropological and nursing perspectives were blended.

The combined nursing and anthropological inquiry into care and cure phenomena provided Leininger with the knowledge base to develop concepts, hypotheses, and other building blocks for the theory of cultural care. Leininger (1988a) writes:

> It took time and in-depth study to link culture and care into a meaningful relationship. The theory of cultural care diversity and universality was difficult to formulate because there was so much to understand about cultures in the world and nursing's perspectives of cultural phenomena. (p. 153)

Because so few nurses were prepared in both anthropology and nursing, Leininger tackled much of this inquiry and theory development on her own (Leininger, 1980; 1984a; 1988a; 1989a; 1991b). Her recognition that there was a lack of nurses prepared for such a challenge and her beliefs that "patients have a *right* to have their sociocultural backgrounds understood" (Leininger, 1970, pp. 45-46) led her to develop courses and programs in what came to be known as transcultural (or crosscultural) nursing (Leininger, 1984b).

Leininger writes that she is frequently asked what has most influenced her theoretical thinking. To these queries she replies

> I would have to answer, rather candidly, that there was no one person or philosophic school of thought, or ideology, *per se*, that directly influenced my thinking. I developed the theory by working on the potential interrelationships of *culture* and *care* through creative think-

ing and by philosophizing from my past professional nursing experiences and anthropological insights . . . (Leininger, 1991, p. 20)

Ideas and themes related to the development and refinement of
the theory of culture care are found in virtually all of her publications. As a prolific writer, Leininger has authored articles, book
chapters, and books focusing on a number of subjects—most of
which are related through ideas about cultural care. Topics for which
Leininger is most well known are the theory of culture care, care and
caring concepts, transcultural nursing concepts, and qualitative research methods.

## Evolution of the Theory

Components of the theory of culture care diversity and universality and the sunrise model have been under development for over 3
decades. Leininger recently commented that she knows of at least 10
versions of her model. Although there are many versions of the
model, there are fewer publications that address the theory as a
whole. Two major articles that present Leininger's theory of cultural
care were published in 1985 and 1988. A book outlining the theory
and its research applications was published in 1991. Thus rigorous
preparatory work in concept analysis and model development have
been Leininger's focus in preparation for the presentation of the
ideas in theory form.

### Concept Development

Development of the concepts of care and caring was a necessary
first step in the evolution of Leininger's theory. Therefore more of
Leininger's publications have been directed toward describing aspects of these concepts than have been directed toward describing
either the sunrise model or theory of culture care. Understanding
the history of Leininger's ideas pertaining to the concepts of care
and caring is, therefore, crucial to understanding her model and
theory.

As early as 1970, Leininger identified the words *care* and *caring* in
a major publication as important nursing elements. These components of nursing were chosen by Leininger for discussion in a book

chapter describing the nature of nursing and how nursing and anthropology could complement each other. *Care* was first defined as a noun that implied "the provision of personalized and necessary services to help man maintain his health state or recover from illness" (Leininger, 1970, p. 30). *Caring* was the verb counterpart to the noun and Leininger believed it implied "a feeling of compassion, interest, and concern for people" (Leininger, 1970, p. 30). This publication not only signaled Leininger's focus on care in nursing but also on the importance of the separation of the concepts "care" and "caring" for fuller understanding. This separation remains a theme throughout the rest of Leininger's writings to the present day. Definitions of these concepts have continued to evolve over time.

By the mid 1970s, Leininger began the development of ideas about the dichotomy between caring and curing. Caring was viewed as the most critical component of curing consequences (Leininger, 1977). By 1984, Leininger expanded this idea to maintain that there could be no curing without caring but that caring could take place without curing. This theme also remains prevalent in Leininger's writings to the present day.

In the late 1970s, Leininger focused on the differences between caring in a generic and professional sense. Generic care/caring was defined as "those assistive, supportive, or facilitative acts toward or for another individual or group with evident or anticipated needs to ameliorate or improve a human condition or lifeway" (Leininger, 1981b, p. 9). Professional caring was seen as "those cognitive and culturally learned action behaviors, techniques, processes, or patterns that enable (or help) an individual, family, or community to improve or maintain a favorably healthy condition or lifeway" (p. 9). Further, professional nursing care was also defined. It was viewed as "those cognitively learned humanistic and scientific modes of helping or enabling an individual, family, or community to receive personalized services" (p. 9).

Leininger's focus on distinguishing between care/caring as known from the perspective of lay people of the culture with that known by professionals reflects her background in anthropology. In cultural anthropology, a prominent theme is the importance of understanding differences between an emic and an etic view. *Emic* "refers to the language expressions, perceptions, beliefs, and practices of individuals or groups of a particular culture in regard to certain phenomena" (Leininger, 1984c, p. 135). *Etic* "refers to the *universal* language expressions, beliefs, and practices in regard to certain phenomena that pertain to several cultures or groups" (Leininger, 1984c, p. 134). This anthropological theme, then, is a logical basis for Leininger's differentiation between generic and professional care.

In early definitions of generic and professional care, it was only professional care that included the idea that the behaviors, acts, or processes were learned. By the late 1980s Leininger further developed the concept of generic care by identifying the concept of generic care knowledge. The concept was defined as referring "to the *epistemological and theoretically derived sources that characterize the fundamental nature of the human care phenomenon*" (Leininger, 1988b, p. 16). The concept of professional care knowledge was also developed at this time. It referred to "the *application of generic knowledge, by the use of learned professional knowledge about care, in creative and practical ways to alleviate a human condition or to sustain health caring practices*" (Leininger, 1988b, p. 17).

By the early 1980s, Leininger became known as a leading proponent of the idea that nursing was synonymous with caring. This was evidenced in statements such as "caring is the central, unique, dominant, and unifying focus of nursing" (1984c, p. 92) and "caring is nursing" (Leininger 1984c, p. 83). These themes remain prominent in Leininger's writings to the present day.

Paralleling concerns emerging in nursing about the value of, and contrast between, subjective and objective knowledge, Leininger found it useful to distinguish between humanistic caring and scientific caring. She proposed that humanistic caring be given as much attention as scientific aspects of caring. Humanistic caring was characterized as "*the subjective feelings, experiences, and interactional behaviors between two or more persons (or groups)* in which assistive or enabling acts are performed generally without prior sets of verified or tested knowledge" (Leininger, 198lc, p. 101). Scientific caring differed in that it was thought to be "*tested activities and judgments in assisting an individual or group,* based upon verified and quantified knowledge related to specific variables" (Leininger, 1981c, p. 101).

The identification of care diversities and care universals was another concern of Leininger. She defined transcultural nursing as comparative caring (Leininger, 1981a). In order to compare caring, it was important that nurses learn culturally congruent care/caring ideas and analyze the similarities and differences in care/caring between or among cultures. This theme remains prominent in Leininger's writings to the present day and is the basis for the title of her theory, culture care diversity and universality.

Culture care diversity "refers to the variabilities and/or differences in meanings, patterns, values, lifeways, or symbols of care within or between collectivities that are related to assistive, supportive, and facilitative, or enabling human care expressions" (Leininger, 1991a, p. 47). Cultural care universality "refers to the common, similar, or dominant uniform care meanings, patterns, values, lifeways, or symbols that are manifest among many cultures and reflect assistive, supportive, facilitative, or enabling ways to help people, another individual, or group that are derived from a specific culture to improve or ameliorate a human condition or lifeway" (Leininger, 1991a, p. 47).

Leininger further developed the concepts of care and caring by describing ethnocaring and cultural care. Ethnocaring referred "to *emic* cognitive assistive, facilitative, or enabling acts or decisions that are valued and practiced to help individuals, families, or groups" (Leininger, 1984c, p. 135). Cultural care was defined as "the subjectively and objectively learned and transmitted values, beliefs, and patterned lifeways that assist, support, facilitate, or enable another individual or group to maintain their well-being and health, to improve their human condition and lifeway, or to deal with illness, handicaps, or death" (Leininger, 1991a, p. 47). The concepts of "ethnocaring" and "cultural care" are very closely related and at times may be used interchangeably.

Other concepts that Leininger clarified by adding the prefix ethno- include ethnohealth, ethnonursing, and ethnohistory (Leininger, 1984c; 1991a). The term *cultural* is used as an adjective in many of Leininger's concepts. Examples are cultural care diversity, cultural care universality, cultural care accommodation, cultural care preservation, cultural care repatterning and new cultural care practices.

Leininger developed the concepts of care and caring by analyzing them within new contexts and in the face of new trends emerging in the disciplines of both anthropology and nursing. A recent example of this is Leininger's (1990a) concern with ethical culture care and her description of four contextual spheres of ethical and moral care (personal or individual, professional or group, institutional or community, and cultural or societal). Leininger wants nurses to understand that ethical and moral aspects "are *culturally constituted and expressed* within meaningful living contexts" (1990a, p. 64).

## Model Development

Leininger is well known for the sunrise model (depicted in this book in Chapter 2). This model first appeared in a major publication in 1984 in the book *Care: The Essence of Nursing and Health*. A few prominent early models contributing to the development of the sunrise model are reviewed here.

In 1976 Leininger presented what she called a transcultural health model. It was described as a "structural functional culture-based model" in that it included major social and cultural factors influencing health care systems. The model was designed to provide a guide for the study and analysis of the major variables found within different cultures in order to obtain a "transcultural health care perspective of health-illness systems" (Leininger, 1976, p. 17).

The 1976 model consisted of two major components: levels of analysis and major domains of study and analysis. Four major levels of analysis and corresponding domains of study were suggested. Level I was analysis of social structure features and the domains associated with the level were political, economic, social (including kinship), cultural (including religion), technological, educational, demographic, and environment factors. Level II was analysis of cultural values and health care. The domains associated with this level of analysis were dominant cultural values and health care values. Level III was analysis of health care systems and typologies. Major domains of study associated with this level included folk and professional health systems. Level IV analysis focused on roles and functions of health professionals. Domains of study included role responsibility and functions.

In 1978 Leininger presented another model for use in studying transcultural and ethnocaring concepts building upon the 1976 work. The 1978 model, published in the 1981 book, *Caring: An Essential Human Need*, contained three phases as follows:

I. Major souces of ethnocaring
II. Classification of ethnocaring and nursing care constructs
III. Analysis and testing of constructs and use of findings (Leininger, 1981b).

In Phase I analysis, the general ethnography of lifeways, major social structure features, cultural values, and health illness caring system ("including beliefs, values, norms, and role caring practices") are examined (Leininger, 1981b, p. 13). Phase II involves learning and classifying care concepts. Phase III consists of analysis of major ethnocaring constructs, theoretical formulations, research testing of the theory, anaysis of ethnocaring research data, and determining nursing interventions based upon research findings (Leininger, 1981b).

In 1979 Leininger offered what she called a "multilevel conceptual model for caring" (Leininger, 1981c, p. 99). This model was developed to "conceptualize and analyze the scope, nature, and structures of caring phenomenon [sic]" (Leininger, 1981c, p. 99). Once again, the model contains levels of analysis corresponding to levels of abstraction. It depicts six levels of caring phenomena: those of the individual, family or social group, the institution or system, specific culture, the societal focus, and the world-wide or multicultural focus. World-wide and societal levels represent the highest level of abstraction, specific culture and institutional levels represent the mid-level of abstraction, and family or social group and individual focus represent the lowest level of abstraction. Leininger maintains that "the interplay and interrelationships among *all* levels of the model are important for a complete analysis of caring" (1981c, p. 100).

In 1980, Leininger described a "taxonomy model to study types of care phenomenon" (1981d, p.137). In this article, Leininger referred to the 1978 model (described above) as helping nurses "conceptualize, order, and study types of caring phenomenon" (1981d, p. 137). Leininger's contribution to the further development of the model in this work is the proposal of a suggested taxonomy of care/caring. The taxonomy of care/caring constructs presented in 1980 builds on Phase II of the 1978 model. Leininger's taxonomy is categorized as follows:

    I. Universal care types and attributes
   II. Cultural specific care types and attributes
  III. Transcultural emic-etic care relationships
  IV. Health professional and nonprofessional care attributes
   V. Social structure and individual group/care types and relationships
  VI. Transcultural nursing care by specific cultures

VII. Interdisciplinary care types

VIII. Other types of care and relation to cure types (Leininger, 1981d, p. 142).

Since 1984, Leininger has consistently represented her model as the Leininger sunrise model. The model has been variously described as a theoretic and conceptual model that depicts transcultural dimensions for "culturologic interviews, assessments, and therapy goals" (Leininger, 1984c, p. 137), a "differential conceptual theoretical and research method to study diversity and universality of care phenomena" (Leininger, 1985b, p. 44), "a conceptual picture to depict components of the theory to study how these components influence care and health status of individuals, families, groups and sociocultural institutions" (Leininger, 1988a, p. 156), and "a valuable cognitive map to guide researchers" (Leininger, 1991a, p. 53).

Leininger explains that the model assists readers to keep "in mind the total gestalt of diverse influences to describe and explain care with health and well being outcomes" (1991a, p. 50). As such, it serves as a safeguard against viewing salient cultural dimensions as fragmented parts.

The model is likened by Leininger to a culture because it "has wholeness and interrelatedness with the nature of the full connections to be studied in relation to human care" (1991a, p. 50). It is designed to help nurses "envision a cultural world of different life forces or influencers on human conditions which need to be considered to discover human care in its fullest ways" (Leininger, 1991a, p. 50).

## Theory Development

Numerous premises, assumptions, and hypotheses describing the nature of cultural care have been presented over the years by Leininger. Two major articles and one book fully address her theory; the articles were published in 1985 and 1988, the book in 1991.

In 1985, Leininger presents what she calls a general theory statement. She writes "with the theory, I predict that different cultures perceive, know, and practice care in different ways, yet there are some commonalities about care among all the cultures in the world" (1985a, p. 4). This is the core of the theory of care diversity and universality from a transcultural viewpoint. Moreover, Leininger (1985a) states that the theory

> explains and predicts human care patterns of cultures and nursing care practices. It can explain and predict factors that influence care, health, and nursing care. Folk, professional, and nursing care values, beliefs, and practices as well as institutional norms, can be identified and explained by the theory. (p. 210)

In the 1985 description, the theory is referred to as "the theory of transcultural care diversity and universality" (Leininger, 1985a, p. 209). In the 1988 article, Leininger refers to the work as "the nursing theory of cultural care diversity and universality" (1988a, p. l52). The word transcultural has been replaced with cultural in the latest publications.

Leininger's 1985 representation of the theory contained a description of 10 concepts, 13 assumptions, and 14 relational statements. The 1988 version included 8 assumptions, 15 definitions, and no explicit relational statements. Most of the changes in the latter publication reflect a synthesis or reformulation of elements found in the 1985 work. The 1991 version of the theory contained definitions of 18 concepts, 13 assumptions, and no explicit relational statements.

It should be noted that Leininger prefers the use of the word construct instead of concept in discussing components of her theory and research findings. She writes "construct is a much broader and more inclusive term than concept, for it has many implicit and explicit meanings that have to be teased out in research processing" (1991a, p. 63).

Leininger maintains that care is the central concept for nursing theory and research. In promoting this idea she questions the very foundation that many nurses accept as the basis for their discipline and profession. For example, Leininger questions the themes of focus for nursing enquiry presented by Donaldson and Crowley (1978) and also states "the four proclaimed concepts of health, nursing, person, and environment . . . seem no longer acceptable" (1991a, p. 59). She states that care is the major metaparadigm or core nursing concept, believing that there are numerous inadequacies with the concepts of health, nursing, person, and environment as major dimensions of nursing.

Leininger does not believe that the concepts of nursing and person (adopted by other nurse theorists as core concepts) can help to explain nursing. She maintains that "one cannot explain nor predict the same phenomenon one is studying" and "nursing is the phenomenon to be explained" (1988a, p. 154). The concept of person "is not sufficient to explain nursing as it fails to account for groups, families, social institutions, and cultures" (Leininger, 1988a, p. 154), and many non-Western cultures do not believe in or focus on the concept of person (Leininger, 1991). Leininger acknowledges the importance of the concepts of environment and health to nursing but notes that these concepts are not unique to nursing since they are studied by other disciplines.

Another area in which Leininger differs from many nurses is in her definition of theory. In 1988, Leininger presented a definition of theory as "sets of interrelated knowledge with meanings and experiences that describe, explain, predict, or account for some phenomenon (or domain of inquiry) through an open, creative, and naturalistic discovery process" (1988a, p. 154). The theory of cultural care fits this definition.

Leininger's definition varies from the classic characterization of theory. It was designed by Leininger to encourage research and the discovery of care phenomena that might be stifled by rigid adherence to other scientific methods. Leininger promotes the use of qualitative research methods in explaining and predicting care phenomena.

## Future Theory Development

Leininger predicts a greater interest in her theory in the future as a result of market forces affecting nursing such as desire for personalized care services and the promotion of quality care as a product (Leininger, 1988b). The theory is thought to be "the broadest and most wholistic guide to study human beings with their lifeways, cultural values and beliefs, symbols, material and nonmaterial forms, and living contexts" (Leininger, 1988a, p. 155).

Future market and societal forces combined with a broad view make the theory desirable and potentially applicable to a wide range of cultures, problems, and nursing situations. As the theory is used by nurses in practice and in research it will be further refined.

Future work might focus on the area of further outlining relationships between components of the theory. For example, Tripp-Reimer and Dougherty (1985) believe that "assumptions on which the model are based are not separated from the theoretical statements" (p. 79).

Leininger continues to refine and develop the theory through application in research examining care values and practices of differing cultural groups. Numerous nurses in the United States and around the world are contributing to these efforts.

## Summary

The theory of cultural care diversity and universality developed by Madeleine Leininger has its roots in both anthropology and nursing. Leininger maintains that culture and care are inextricably linked and that care/caring is the central concern of nurses. The goal of Leininger's theoretical works is to provide culturally congruent nursing care.

Leininger has been involved in concept, model, and theory development for over 3 decades. As a result, the concept of care has been analyzed in many different ways in Leininger's writings. Examples of this analysis include the definition and comparison of the terms care and caring, generic and professional care, and humanistic care and scientific care. Numerous early models have led to the well-known Leininger sunrise model of our current day.

The theory of culture care diversity and universality has as its core idea that there are differences and similarities in care among all cultures of the world. The theory is different from the model in that the model only depicts components of the theory to provide a conceptual picture. The theory was originally known as the theory of transcultural diversity and universality but more recently the prefix trans- has been dropped. Concept, model, and theory development efforts are continuing.

# 2

---

## *Assumptive Premises of the Theory*

MADELEINE M. LEININGER

Making assumptive premises about a theory is important; indeed, they can be considered as the basic "givens" of a theory. Initially, I wondered what could be the relationship of nursing care to culture, and I came to believe that care was dependent upon culture, and culture could not survive without care. Hence, culture was critical and essential to understand people and nursing.

I am continually examining assumptions about the theory and how the theory could generate fresh knowledge in nursing. The assumptions below (Leininger, 1991a, pp. 44-45) came from thinking inductively and deductively and from readings and experiences in nursing and anthropology. They have been refined over the past 3 decades, but they are major ideas that guided my deliberations in developing the theory of cultural care.

1. Care is the essence of nursing and a distinct, dominant, central, and unifying focus.
2. Care (caring) is essential for well-being, health, healing, growth, survival, and facing handicaps or death.

3. Culture care is the broadest holistic means to know, explain, interpret, and predict nursing care phenomena to guide nursing care practices.

4. Nursing is a transcultural humanistic and scientific care discipline and profession with the central purpose to serve human beings worldwide.

5. Care (caring) is essential to curing and healing, for there can be no curing without caring.

6. Culture care concepts, meanings, expressions, patterns, processes, and structural forms of care have different (diversity) and similar (towards commonalities or universalities) characteristics among all cultures of the world.

7. Every human culture has generic (lay, folk, or indigenous) care knowledge and practices and usually professional care knowledge and practices, which vary transculturally.

8. Cultural care values, beliefs, and practices are influenced by and tend to be embedded in world view, language, religion (or spiritual), kinship (social), politics (or legal), education, economic, technology, ethnohistory, and environmental context of a particular culture.

9. Beneficial, healthy, and satisfying culturally-based nursing care contributes to the well-being of individuals, families, groups, and communities within their environmental context.

10. Culturally congruent nursing care can only occur when culture care values, expressions, or patterns are known and used appropriately and meaningfully by the nurse with individuals or groups.

11. Culture care differences and similarities between professional caregivers and clients (with their generic needs) exist in human cultures worldwide.

12. Clients who show signs of culture conflicts, noncompliance, stresses, and ethical or moral concerns need nursing care that is culturally-based.

13. The qualitative paradigm with naturalistic inquiry modes provides the essential means to discover human care transculturally.

These assumptive premises guided and stimulated my thinking as I systematically developed and studied the theory of culture care with the ethnonursing, ethnoscience, and ethnographic methods.

The assumptions served as a springboard for my theoretical understandings, hunches, and predictions about culture care.

## Orientational Definitions of the Theory

In order to develop fully the theory of culture care, I realized that I had to have *orientational concepts* or *constructs*. Thus I developed the idea of orientational definitions (or ballpark ideas), which was in contrast to *operational definitions* (a very tightly constructed ballpark idea).

In the early 1980s a small group of nurse leaders proposed four nursing concepts: nursing, person, health, and environment (Fawcett, 1984, 1989; Fitzpatrick & Whall, 1989). In my work, I had already focused on care as central to nursing, and culture and environmental context as critical to nursing, yet the concept of care was missing from their concepts, and culture was never identified. I found some of the concepts inadequate to explain, predict, and know nursing. First, I felt nursing could not be explained in terms of nursing itself; a theorist needs to use different ideas to discover the nature of a phenomenon. Second, from a social science perspective, *person* has a specific definition—someone with a particular status and social role. And it would be inapproriate to focus only on the person as central to nursing because nurses function with families, groups, communities, and institutions.

I believed the concept of "environment" could be important to nursing because nurses function in many different kinds of environments, but I did not view it as central. In the development of the theory, I had already defined and used the term *environmental context*, a much broader concept. I saw this term refer to the totality of human existence in different kinds of sociocultural and psychophysical environments. Thus environment had a much broader meaning and referred to holism—or the totality of human living.

The concept of "health," is important, but I found it limiting as defined by the theorists. From my transcultural studies, I had discovered that well-being and other phenomena were closely related to or used interchangeably with health.

Today, it is encouraging to witness the increased focus on human "care" and "caring," and to see more nurses study and value care as the central and most important phenomenon of nursing (Gaut, 1981; Leininger, 1981a, 1981b, 1984a, 1984b, 1984c, 1988a, 1988b, 1988c, 1988d, 1990a, 1990b, 1991a, 1991b; Ray, 1981; Valentine, 1988; Watson, 1985). In fact, there has been a groundswell of interest in human care as the central focus of nursing education and practice in the last decade. The focus on human care with culture has stimulated many nurses to obtain a more complete and holistic view of nursing.

Another unique feature in developing the culture care theory was mainly the use of an inductive research method called ethnonursing to define and discover culture care. The theory was developed from the qualitative paradigm or perspective in order to tease out the meanings, understanding, characteristics, and attributes of culture care from the people's local viewpoints or the emic views (Leininger, 1978, 1985b), a markedly different approach from the traditional quantitative paradigm in which researchers focus on testing hypotheses and specific variables that are predetermined and interesting mainly to the researcher and not necessarily to those being studied. With the qualitative paradigm, the researcher uses "orientational" rather than "operational" definitions. The latter definitions are used with the "quantitative paradigm." Orientational definitions facilitate an open discovery way to uncover phenomena or a broad domain of inquiry. This approach in theory development and study is important because it permits the local people's viewpoints, ideas, and experiences to come forth and because it contrasts sharply with "etic" or the researcher's viewpoints and helps the research to enter the informant's world. Orientational definitions might change according to what the reseacher discovers. I also used the term *construct*, which refers to many embedded ideas or concepts "within" a term, whereas *concept* is a single idea or phenomenon.

The major orientational definitions for the theory are (Leininger, 1991a, pp. 46-47):

1.  *Care* (noun) refers to abstract and concrete phenomena related to assisting, supporting, or enabling experiences or behaviors toward or for others with evident or anticipated needs to ameliorate or improve a human condition or lifeway.
2.  *Caring* (gerund) refers to actions and activities directed toward assisting, supporting, or enabling another individual or group

with evident or anticipated needs to ameliorate or improve a human condition or lifeway, or to face death.

3. *Culture* refers to the learned, shared, and transmitted values, beliefs, norms, and lifeways of a particular group that guides their thinking, decisions, and actions in patterned ways.

4. *Culture care* refers to the cognitively learned and transmitted values, beliefs, and patterned lifeways that assist, support, facilitate, or enable another individual or group to maintain their well-being or health, to improve their human condition and lifeway, or to deal with illness, handicaps, or death.

5. *Health* refers to a state of well-being that is culturally defined, valued, and practiced, and that reflects the ability of individuals (or groups) to perform their daily role activities in culturally expressed, beneficial, and patterned lifeways.

6. *Environmental context* refers to the totality of an event, situation, or particular experiences that give meaning to human expressions, interpretations, and social interactions in particular physical, ecological, sociopolitical and/or cultural settings.

7. *Cultural care diversity* refers to the variabilities and/or differences in meanings, patterns, values, lifeways, or symbols of care within or between collectivities that are related to assistive, supportive, or enabling human care expressions.

8. *Cultural care universality* refers to the common, similar, or dominant uniform care meanings, patterns, values, lifeways, or symbols that are manifest among many cultures and reflect assistive, supportive, facilitative, or enabling ways to help people. (The term *universality* is not used in an absolute way nor as a fixed statistical finding).

9. *Generic folk or lay system* refers to culturally learned and transmitted, indigenous (or traditional), folk (home-based) knowledge and skills used to provide assistive, supportive, enabling, or facilitative acts toward or for another individual, group, or institution with evident or anticipated needs to ameliorate or improve a human lifeway, health condition (or well-being), or to deal with handicaps and death situations.

10. *Professional system(s)* refers to formal and cognitively learned professional knowledge and practice skills that are taught in professional institutions to a number of multidisciplinary personnel in order to serve consumers seeking health services.

11. *Cultural care preservation or maintenance* refers to those assistive, supportive, facilitative, or enabling professional actions and decisions that help people of a particular culture to retain and/or

preserve relevant care values so that they can maintain their well-being, recover from illness, or face handicaps and/or death.

12. *Culture care accommodation or negotiation* refers to those assistive, supportive, facilitative, or enabling creative professional actions and decisions that help people of a designated culture to adapt to, or to negotiate with, others for a beneficial or satisfying health outcome with professional care providers.

13. *Cultural care repatterning or restructuring* refers to those assistive, supportive, facilitative, or enabling professional actions and decisions that help clients reorder, change, or modify their lifeways for new, different, or more beneficial health care patterns while respecting the client's cultural values and beliefs and providing a better (or healthier) lifeway than before.

14. *Cultural congruent (nursing) care* refers to those cognitively based assistive, supportive, facilitative, or enabling acts or decisions that are tailor-made to fit with an individual's, group's, or institution's cultural values, beliefs, and lifeways in order to provide meaningful, beneficial, and satisfying health care, or well-being services.

*Other Orientational Definitions*
*(Leininger, 1991a)*

1. *Nursing* refers to a learned humanistic and scientific profession and discipline that is focused on human care phenomena and activities in order to assist, support, facilitate, or enable individuals or groups to maintain or regain their well-being (or health) in culturally meaningful and beneficial ways, or to help people face handicaps or death.

2. *World view* refers to the way people tend to look out upon the world or their universe to form a picture or a value stance about their life or world around them.

3. *Cultural and social structure dimensions* refer to the dynamic patterns and features of interrelated structural and organizational factors of a particular culture (subculture or society), which includes religious, kinship (social), political (and legal), economic, educational, technologic, and cultural values, and how these factors may be interrelated and function to influence human behavior in different environmental contexts.

4. *Ethnohistory* refers to those past facts, events, instances, and experiences of individuals, groups, cultures, and institutions that

are primarily people-centered (ethno) and that describe, explain, and interpret human lifeways within particular cultural contexts and space-time referents.

The above orientational definitions serve as guideposts to discover phenomena bearing upon culture care. These definitions orient the theorist and researcher to explore general ideas under study with the ethnonursing research method—a method explicitly designed to study culture care theory (Leininger, 1991a). The ethnonursing method was developed to tease out culture care meanings, expressions, and patterns bearing upon nursing, because culture care was usually lodged or embedded in the social structure and language uses. Quantitative methods are extremely difficult to use to study covert and complex culture care meanings and expressions such as compassion, hope, empathy, and many other constructs. A researcher could study culture care from both quantitative and qualitative paradigms; however, one must remember *not* to mix the paradigms as this would be violating the philosophy, purposes, and goals of each paradigm (Leininger, 1990b, 1991a; Lincoln & Guba, 1985).

## Essential Features of the Culture Care Theory

Because a researcher needs to discover and explicate meanings, expressions, and patterns of culture care from different cultures, I needed an inductive theory and thus defined theory as *patterns or sets of interrelated concepts, constructs, expressions, meanings, and experiences that describe, explain, predict, and account for some phenomena or domain of inquiry through an open, creative, and naturalistic discovery process* (Leininger, 1991a, p. 34). This definition of a theory would facilitate studying culture care using a naturalistic discovery process and lead to in-depth descriptions, as well as ways to understand, explain, interpret, and even predict nursing phenomena through patterns and themes. My theory definition is similar to Steven's (1979) and Watson's (1985), which focus on discovery describing and interpreting phenomena as fully as possible. An inductive-based theory allows for thick descriptive data from informants, situations, events, instances, and groups and from environmental contexts to be uncovered by the researcher. Teasing out covert and complex phenomena requires considerable attention to the people's values and lifeways. Making interpretations from informants' ideas are important, as is documenting the context being studied. Thus these broad and open definitions were essential to tap unknown areas, to get data directly from the people to understand culture care phenomena, and to examine the assumptive premises of the theory.

In developing the theory of culture care, I wanted to consider what is universal and diverse about culture care worldwide. A broad theoretical perspective was essential to study cultural care variations and similarities among and between cultures of the world. The theory was, therefore, very broad in scope, with a worldwide perspective. I was curious if there were patterns, meanings, and practices of care that were universal or common, because this knowledge would help nurses as they cared for people in different cultures. At the same time, I was curious about what was diverse or different about care. Discovering the universals (or commonalities) and differences (diversities) was essential to establish a foundation of nursing knowledge. Nurses could use findings from the theory in practical ways to improve or provide nursing care that was meaningful and culturally sensitive to the client's needs. Such discoveries would be an entirely new breakthrough in nursing and provide new knowledge to nurses.

The theory was envisioned and developed so that it could be used in our Western world, such as the United States, Canada, and Europe, and also in non-Western cultures, such as China, Korea, South Africa, and other places. Comparative data about human care was essential to provide differential care to clients and to make decisions and actions about the nursing care that fit clients' needs. Over time, the theory focused on where nursing was practiced or needed to be practiced in the future based on the people's needs and desires. Thus the theory was designed to have very useful and practical outcomes and to be used to provide culturally sensitive and competent care.

The *purpose* of culture care theory was to discover, through open naturalistic inquiry, culture care diversities and universality in order to generate nursing knowledge for the discipline and profession of nursing. The *goal* of the theory was ultimately to provide "culturally congruent nursing care" in order to improve nursing care to people of different or similar cultures. The latter meant helping clients, through culturally based care, to recover favorably from illness, or to prevent conditions that would limit the client's health or well-being. The goal was, therefore, to provide "culturally congruent" and "culturally specific" nursing care that would lead to health or well-being. Nursing care needed to be tailored to or to fit the clients' cultural values, beliefs, and lifeways. Providing culturally congruent care to individuals, families, groups, or cultures meant that nursing care actions and decisions needed to be beneficial, satisfying, and/or meaningful to the sick, well, or disabled and to help the dying person. I theorized that if nursing care was not culturally congruent a host of conflicts and problems would occur that would delay recovery, prevent wellness, or could even lead to unexpected death. For example, the idea of "protective care" to the elderly in the community could have unfavorable consequences if protective care of the elderly was not valued by that culture.

In theorizing further about culture care, I held to the belief that humanistic care was important and was different from scientific and technical care. Humanistic care was a central and a distinct feature to characterize and identify nursing as a profession and discipline. The term, *essence*, in nursing meant that which makes nursing "that it is," and is an essential feature of how it becomes manifest and expressed to others. "Nursing was held to be caring" and "caring was essential and a dominant feature of nursing" (Leininger, 1981a, 1984a, 1988a). Moreover, nursing needed to be known to consumers and the public at large from both scientific and humanistic perspectives. Discovering differences and similarities between scientific and humanistic viewpoints was a research goal. From my clinical and research experiences, I had already discovered some of the meanings and patterns of care as being compassion, presence, enabling, and many other caring expressions. These discoveries revealed that there is still much more to learn about caring. Competent care is what people seek and expect when ill, but it is also needed to maintain their state of wellness.

I had several predictions about culture care that greatly stimulated my thinking. I predicted that nurses could discover largely unknown, covert, or taken-for-granted features about nursing care modes as they studied different cultures in the world in-depth. New insights about culture care could transform nursing education and practice in the future. This body of new knowledge would be viewed as the "new nursing and discipline knowledge" to guide nurses' actions, decisions, and judgments. Such knowledge was predicted to lead to very different practices from the present-day medical disease and symptoms model. How different cultures perceived and knew of care from their viewpoint and cultural needs was important new knowledge. It was this largely hidden and unknown culture care knowledge that would lead nurses to develop many different kinds of care practices and new understandings that would benefit clients. Such care patterns and practices were *mainly "rooted"* or *grounded in culture values, language, and social structures*. Nurses could no longer treat all clients alike because of cultural variabilities and different care expectations. Cultural diversities and similarities of knowledge of Western and non-Western cultures would lead nurses to value the importance of culture-specific care.

From the beginning I theorized that care was an "essential human need" to help people keep healthy, grow, and function (Leininger, 1980, 1981a, 1981c). Human beings in any culture had to learn about caring attitudes and practices in order to survive in the past and today. Most important, human caring was learned and transmitted to others. *Being human was to be caring, and caring was culturally based.* Caring for others or self required using culturally learned and transmitted values of care, primarily from one's family or cultural group. Healthy people, I held, had learned good caring patterns that kept them well or healthy. In contrast, unhealthy patterns of caring led to illness, disability, and even death. I also held there were *"caring cultures"* where people in organizational structures knew how to care for people. Where beneficial caring patterns and experiences existed, there were healthy caring people. In contrast, noncaring patterns and cultures, I predicted, would lead to illnesses, deaths, or a host of unhealthy conditions (Leininger, 1988a, 1991a). Moreover, the well-being of individuals, families, and specific cultures would be threatened by noncaring expressions, resulting in cultural violence, destruction, and death. Caring patterns were held to be essential to keep people well and to live satisfying and meaningful lives.

These ideas led me to theorize about differences between *generic* and *professional caring.* I conceptualized that there were two kinds of caring that existed in every culture and that needed to be discovered as they had not been identified for their comparative uses in nursing (Leininger, 1970, 1978, 1981a, 1991a). Generic caring was the oldest form and basic expression of human caring essential for the growth, health, and survival of homo sapiens. Generic care as the foundational prototype of care included local home remedies and folk care.

It was predicted all families or housholds had some forms of generic or basic caring that was used by family members or by special caregivers. These generic caring behaviors or expectations needed to be identified for their efficacy or beneficial outcomes and used with professional care practices where indicated. If beneficial generic care were not practiced, one could predict "noncaring" outcomes such as poor recovery from illness, failure to stay well, and other problems. It would be helpful for nurses to know some families with special caregiving and care-recipient practices in home and institutional hospital care. Hence generic care was a new construct conceptualized as important to the theory of culture care and especially in relationship to professional care practices.

*Professional care* was conceptualized to be different from generic care in that professional care was defined as cognitively learned, practiced, and transmitted knowledge learned through formal and informal professional education nursing schools (Leininger, 1991a, p. 34). When nursing students entered nursing, they were taught about professional nursing techniques, practices, and related topics that constituted fundamentals of nursing. Students were expected to learn what constituted professional care or nursing care practices. In some nursing schools, nursing care was often about procedures and practices or ways to handle medical diseases and symptoms. Professional nursing content was often directed toward carrying out aseptic medical techniques, or the "right ways" to be an effective, competent, or skilled nurse in "psychomotor" nursing practices. Professional care also included learning about communication techniques, interpersonal relationships, ethical aspects, and other content held important by nursing leaders. Professional nursing did not include ideas about folk care since it was largely unrecognized and not valued as useful to nursing. With the advent of transcultural nursing, professional and generic care began to be valued and studied.

In theorizing about generic and professional care, I predicted that generic care as naturalistic local, folk, and familiar home care practices would differ considerably from professional care due to cultural factors. If professional and generic care practices did not reasonably fit together, this would influence client recovery, health, and well-being. To provide culturally congruent care, professional and generic care needed to be considered to facilitate meaningful care practices. Thus the ultimate goal was to link and synthesize generic and professional care knowledge to benefit the client. But before this could occur, nurse researchers needed to explicate and know the differences and similarities between the two types of care. This would be extremely important in order to provide culturally congruent care, which I held was essential for quality nursing care practices. I speculated that world view, social structure, language, ethnohistory, and environmental context as defined above would greatly influence both generic and professional care beliefs and practices. Cultural values, religious beliefs, economic concerns, attitudes about technology, kinship ties, educational interests, and world view would impact upon caring methods and, ultimately, the health or well-being of clients. Knowledge of generic and professional care of individuals, families, groups, institutions, and communities was essential to provide professional nursing care.

In order to help nurses visualize components of the theory influencing human care, I developed the sunrise model (see Figure 2.1), a depiction of the components and conceptual areas of the theory that need to be considered in the discovery of factors that influenced generic and professional care practices, which develop culturally congruent nursing care. The model symbolically portrays a rising sun. If nurses systematically examined the conceptual components in the model, they would discover human care and the influence on the health and well-being of individuals, families, communities, and institutions and become enlightened by these findings. The model conceptually depicts the world view, religion, kinship, cultural values, economics, technology, language, ethnohistory, and environmental factors that are predicted to explain and influence culture care. Thus it serves as a cognitive orientation to obtain a complete, holistic, and comprehensive way to examine the theory. Discovering the meanings, and expressive factors of culture care and its potential influence on care and the health or well-being of clients is crucial to the theory. The sunrise model is truly a holistic model that the nurse researcher needs to use as a guide to study the theoretical predictions or hunches made by the theorist. If these different factors were not studied, the nurse would have only partial, fragmented, and inadequate knowledge about culture care. With the use of the sunrise model, the nurse assesses all aspects, including generic folk and professional systems, which give clues to theoretical ways of devel-

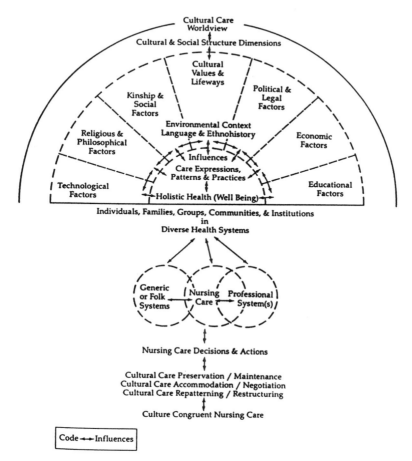

**Figure 2.1.** Leininger's Sunrise Model to Depict Theory of Cultural Care Diversity and Universality

SOURCE: From Leininger, M. (Ed.) (1991). *Culture care diversity and universality: A theory of nursing.* New York: National League for Nursing Press. Reprinted by permission.

oping culturally congruent nursing care. Courses in transcultural nursing, anthropology, and health sciences help the nurse researcher to identify and understand the different components depicted in the sunrise model and focus on the tenets of the theory.

The sunrise model reflects my theory about nursing not only as an intellectual discipline, but as a practice profession. Accordingly I theorize that there are "three modes of action or decision" to guide nurses in providing culturally congruent care: *(a) cultural care preservation and/or maintenance, (b) cultural care accommodation and/or negotiation, and (c) cultural care repatterning and restructuring* (Leininger, 1988a, 1991a). These three modes could lead to the goal of the theory, which is to provide culturally congruent nursing care. The nurse would consider data obtained from the informant, from observations, and from the study of all components in the sunrise model to identify which care mode (or modes) would best fit and benefit the client's needs. Data from the sunrise model would guide the nurse to develop creative and appropriate ways to examine the three action or decision modes. From the use of grounded, culturally-based people data, cultural patterns, and culture-specific ideas for congruent nursing care practices would emerge. The wealth of data from the individual or family about their world view, social structure factors, environmental context, and other aspects should reveal fresh and informative modes to guide nursing care practices.

In general, I held with the theory of culture care that there would be some similarities (the commonalities or universalities) along with the differences (diversities) among cultures with regard to culture care meanings, patterns, expressions, functions (uses), structural features, and practices (Leininger, 1988a, 1991b). These similarities and differences needed to be teased out and made known in order to arrive at a holistic perspective of human care with specific cultures. I also postulated that specific care expressions or patterns such as presence, respect, support, enabling, compassion, and many other care constructs could be powerful factors for the nurse to use to help people remained well or healthy (Leininger, 1981a, 1984a, 1991a). I called these care constructs the "golden nuggets" that needed to be fully discovered, valued, and used in order to provide therapeutic and meaningful nursing care practices to culturally diverse clients. These golden nuggets were essential for nurses to help people recover from illnesses, to remain well, or to face dying in a culturally congruent and satisfying way. I predicted that where specific caring meanings and patterns were known and used in nursing, health ways would prevail; if noncaring expressions existed, one would find unfavorable, unhealthy care practices. These culture care constructs were, indeed, the *essence* of what nursing is or should be and were the means to help nurses provide meaningful quality nursing care. Still today, these powerful care constructs of different cultures are slowly being discovered and understood to guide professional nursing education care practices. Nursing with a culture care focus can influence the outcome of professional care practices. Thus culture care theory was a new, comprehensive means to discover embedded care phenomena and to use the knowledge to transform nursing education and practice. Culture care knowledge was much needed to provide specific and differential nursing care practices and to shift current nursing practices from dominant medical emphases to a nursing perspective.

In studying and examining the theory, the *ethnonursing qualitative paradigm research method* proved to be most helpful to tease out and understand culture data and its meanings within nursing contexts. The ethnonursing method has helped nurse researchers to: (a) explicate nursing phenomena about culture care; (b) get emic-grounded data through inductive and naturalistic approaches rather than focusing on the researcher's etic (outsider's) knowledge and interpretations; (c) use different enabling inquiry guides to probe for embedded meanings, interpretations, and relationships among different components of the theory; (d) discover specific details related to the care constructs and ideas related to the theory; (e) identify highly creative ways nurses can use culture care knowledge in client care; (f) show ways nurses can get close to culture-specific ideas about human care; and (g) discover ways to blend professional and generic care knowledge for the benefit of clients from diverse cultures.

## Research Findings

The seven major research studies presented in the *Culture Care Diversity and Universality* theory publication (Leininger, 1991, pp. 73-119) demonstrate the importance of the ethnonursing method and the theory with research findings by Bohay, Gates, Leininger, Rosenbaum, Spangler, Stasiak, and Wenger. I have studied a number of cultures and found culture-specific care values, meanings, and actions from 23 cultures as generated from the theory (Leininger, 1991a, pp. 119-134). These findings are already providing new insights to the practice of nursing.

Because the theory is being used extensively around the world to study multicultural and culture care phenomena, one can predict that it will spread even more in the future. Currently, the theory is being used by nurses in Finland, Sweden, the Middle East, Africa, Japan, Canada, Australia, Europe, Korea, China, South America, Russia, Tibet, and several places in the Pacific Islands. In addition, some nonnurses and other professionals are finding the theory relevant to their work by modifying some terms of theory to fit their discipline uses. Organizational theorists and administrators are excited about the theory because it gives them a broad framework to understand the diverse factors impacting their areas of interest. Corporate executives have told the theorist how much it helped them to study broad areas they needed to include in assessing their administrative goals and caring ethos.

Nurse theorists and researchers will continue to realize the critical importance of the theory as one of the most comprehensive, holistic means to discover human care phenomena. Nurses are realizing the actual and potentially powerful role of culture care that influences nursing practice and education. Culture care as a theoretical synthesis construct also has practical uses to discover, understand, and make decisions about nursing practices, especially with the use of the sunrise model. The theory is being taught in schools of nursing and used as a major conceptual guide for nursing curricula. Culture care provides the "golden nuggets" and many other rich insights for advancing nursing's discipline knowledge. Growing multiculturalism will make it imperative for nurses to function in diverse cultures. Transcultural care research knowledge based on culture care and health will guide nursing decisions and actions. The future for this culture care theory looks exceedingly promising for the discipline and profession of nursing. The next section will reveal some exciting implications for the use of culture care theory in clinical nursing practices and education.

# 3

## The Theory of Culture Care: Implications for Nursing

### CHERYL L. REYNOLDS

The broad scope of the theory of culture care diversity and universality as proposed by Madeleine Leininger makes it useful in many nursing settings and situations. Contributions of the theory to the profession and discipline of nursing can be found in practice, administration, education, and research.

### Nursing Practice

Leininger has very clearly described the way her theory applies to nursing practice. The goal of the theory is to provide culturally congruent nursing care to persons of diverse cultures (Leininger, 1988a). Discovering cultural care/caring beliefs, values, and practices and analyzing the similarities and differences of these beliefs between and among cultures will help nurses attain this goal.

Leininger states that it is important for the nurse to understand the patient's view of illness. This includes "how the patient knows and understands his illness, how he desires to be helped, and the ways health personnel can help him" (Leininger, 1969, p. 2). The Leininger sunrise model portrayed in the book *Care: The Essence of Nursing and Health* is described as a model for culturologic interviews, assessments, and therapy goals (Leininger, 1984a). Thus the model can help nurses develop questions for the assessment of client cultural beliefs related to health and illness. Leininger has also developed a videotape demonstrating major components, techniques, and skills in doing a cultural care assessment of an American-Polish informant.

Few nurse theorists have clearly identified theory-based modes of nursing action that help practitioners understand how to intervene with clients based upon their theory. Leininger has clearly stated ways that nurses can provide culturally congruent care. The dominant modes to guide nursing decisions and actions based upon the theory of cultural care are: (a) cultural care preservation or maintenance, (b) cultural care accomodation or negotiation, and (c) cultural care repatterning or restructuring (Leininger, 1988a).

Cultural care preservation "refers to those assistive, supporting, facilitative, or enabling professional actions and decisions that help people of a particular culture to retain and/or preserve relevant care values so that they can maintain their well-being, recover from illness, or face handicaps and/or death" (Leininger, 1991a, p. 46). Cultural care accomodation "refers to those assistive, supporting, facilitative, or enabling creative professional actions and decisions that help people of a designated culture to adapt to, or to negotiate with, others for a beneficial or satisfying health outcome with professional careproviders" (Leininger, 1991, p. 48). Cultural care repatterning "refers to those assistive, supporting, facilitative, or enabling professional actions and decisions that help a client(s) reorder, change, or greatly modify their lifeways for new, different, and beneficial health care pattern while respecting the client(s) cultural values and beliefs and still providing a beneficial or healthier lifeway than before the changes were coestablished with the client(s) (Leininger, 1991a, p. 49).

In an earlier publication, Leininger (1984b) also identified another mode of nursing action: new cultural care practices. New cultural care practices refer "to the cognitive action of incorporating different or new assistive or facilitative actions designed to be beneficial to the client" (p. 135). This way of acting to promote culturally congruent care has not been addressed in later publications.

It should be noted that Leininger does not characterize her modes of nursing actions as interventions. She maintains that nursing intervention is a Western professional nursing culture-bound term that may communicate to some clients "ideas of cultural interferences and imposition practices" (Leininger, 1991a, p. 55). Moreover, Leininger does not use the terminology "nursing problems" because "all too often the client may not have a problem, or the problem may not be seen as relevant to the people by the nurse" (Leininger, 1991a, p. 55).

Leininger is well known as the founder of the transcultural nursing movement in the United States. The motto of the Transcultural Nursing Society is a quote from Leininger that reads: "That the cultural needs of people in the world will be met by nurses prepared in transcultural nursing."

Transcultural nursing is comparative caring (Leininger, 1981a). It is a "formal area of study and practice of diverse cultures in the world with respect to their care, health and illness values, beliefs, and practices in order to provide culture specific or universal nursing care that is congruent with the client, family, or community's cultural values and lifeways" (Leininger, 1989a, p. 4). Nurses can become certified in this specialty area.

Transcultural nursing is different from international nursing. The term *transcultural* was deliberately chosen by Leininger because it refers to world cultures whether or not they are nationalized, whereas international nursing refers to nationalized cultures only (Leininger, 1991a).

A recent article applying Leininger's theory to intensive care (ICU) nursing practice was published by Kloosterman (1991). The phenomena of sensory alteration frequently encountered in the ICU setting was described by Kloosterman as resulting from culturally incongruent nursing care. Client's unfamiliar with the culture of nursing in the ICU setting became confused when their normal and familiar care patterns were altered.

Leininger has long been concerned with cultural imposition and ethnocentrism on the part of nurses in their daily practice. Awareness of Leininger's theory will help nurses to avoid this problem. While not all transcultural nurses use Leininger's theory as a guide for practice, the Transcultural Nursing Society promotes culturally congruent nursing care in their publications and yearly conferences.

## Nursing Administration

The theory of culture care diversity and universality can be used to analyze the culture of nursing or the culture of an organization just as it can be used in assessment of the individual client. Leininger writes "nurses seldom pause to reflect on how the culture of nursing can influence care practices and attitudes" (1988b, p. 21). The culture of nursing is defined as "those identifiable and inferred normative patterns, values, beliefs, and practices that characterize the profession of nursing over time" (Leininger, 1986, pp. 2-3). This knowledge could be especially important for nurse administrators.

Identifying nurses as members of a cultural group means that it is useful to "examine nurses' cultural values, meanings, and experiences of care so that they can be understood in caregiving experiences" (Leininger, 1986, p. 3). Through analysis of the culture of nursing, Leininger has identified care facilitation and resistance factors inherent in the culture.

Leininger defines care facilitation as "those factors, forces, or conditions that tend to enhance or enable nurses to discover the full meanings and uses of care in their thinking and work" (1986, p. 2). Care resistance is "those factors, forces, or conditions that tend to limit or curtail nurses in the full discovery of the meanings and uses of care" (Leininger, 1986, p. 2).

In describing other ways her theory can be useful in administration, Leininger writes that "from an institutional perspective, it provides a theoretical framework to study how institutions use, interpret, and predict goals that fit with the communities they serve" (1988b, p. 25). Leininger maintains "one can predict the health of an institution by its care beliefs, values, and practices" (1988b, p. 25). In addition, a list of areas of inquiry for nursing service administrators consistent with her theory have been outlined by Leininger (1988b).

Leininger's theory is applicable to the study of organizations and institutions in part because Leininger does not define the singular person as one of the key concepts in the theory. There are many reasons behind Leininger's purposeful omission of this concept, but the main one useful for nursing administrators is that Leininger recognizes that a definition of person "fails to account for groups, families, social institutions, and cultures" (Leininger, 1988a, p. 154).

The theory of culture care diversity and universality is also useful to administrators who are concerned that their institutions deliver quality care to clients of multicultural populations. Nursing administrators with such concerns could use the theory concepts, tenets, and modes of nursing action as means of facilitating the delivery of this care within the organization.

## Nursing Education

Leininger has developed and taught undergraduate and graduate courses in transcultural nursing at the University of Colorado, the University of Washington, the University of Utah, and Wayne State University. She developed doctoral programs in transcultural nursing or with a transcultural nursing emphasis at the University of Washington, the University of Utah, and Wayne State University. These courses and curricula were developed consistent with the theory of cultural care diversity and universality.

By 1980, about 20% of nursing programs accredited by the National League for Nursing incorporated cultural concepts and principles into the undergraduate program (Leininger, 1989b) and by 1991, 15% of graduate nursing programs in the United States had transcultural nursing courses. In 1991, the Transcultural Nursing Society listed five graduate programs in transcultural nursing in the United States and three additional universities where the faculty members are prepared in transcultural nursing and are developing courses on the subject. It is unknown how many nursing programs use Leininger's theory as the basis of their cultural diversity curricula.

Because the theory has direct applicability to nursing practice and research, and because of recent societal and worldwide trends towards increasing travel and respecting cultural diversity, the theory of culture care diversity and universality is useful for nurse educators. In 1986 the American Nurses' Association Council on Cultural Diversity in Nursing Practice stated that "one way to promote an appreciation of various cultures is to develop and implement nursing school curricula that incorporate practice-related concepts of cultural diversity" (p. 1). They also maintain that "nursing education programs must include content in the curriculum pertaining to culturally diverse groups if nurses are to be prepared to provide safe, effective care acceptable to all consumers" (p. 2).

## Research

Application of the theory and model in research was published by Leininger in the study of "Southern Rural Black and White American Lifeways With Focus on Care and Health Phenomena" (1984b; 1985) and a study of "Culture Care of the Gadsup Akuna of the Eastern Highlands of New Guinea" (1991b). Leininger reports that she has also collected and analyzed culture values and culture care themes from 54 cultures. To date she has identified well over 175 care/caring constructs (Leininger, 1991a).

Leininger lists cultural values and culture care meanings and action modes for 23 cultural groups in her book *Culture Care Diversity and Universality: A Theory of Nursing*. The findings include studies of the following cultural groups: Anglo-American, Mexican-American, Haitian-American, African-American, North American Indian, Gadsup Akuna, Phillipine-American, Japanese-American, Vietnamese-American, Southest Indian American, Chinese-American, Arab-American Muslim, Old order Amish-Americans, Appalachian culture, Polish-American culture, German-American culture, Italian-American, Greek-American, Jewish-American, Lithuanian-American, Swedish-American, Finnish-American, and Danish-American.

Numerous graduate and doctoral students have used Leininger's theory as a basis for their research. However, many of these studies are unpublished. Published studies include Wenger and Wenger's study of old order Amish (1988), Gates's (1988) study of caring behaviors experienced by couples during a hysterectomy, Monsma's (1988) study of children of battered women, Rosenbaum's (1988) study of mental health care needs of Soviet-Jewish immigrants, and Luna's (1989) study of transcultural nursing care of Arab Muslims. Research reported in Leininger's 1991 book *Culture Care Diversity and Universality: A Theory of Nursing* includes Bohay's study of culture care meanings and experiences of pregnancy and childbirth of Ukrainians, Gates's study of dying in hospital and hospice contexts, Rosenbaum's study of Greek Canadian widows, Spangler's study of Phillipine and Anglo-American nurses, Stasiak's study of Mexican-American urbanites, and Wenger's study of old order Amish. In addition, Rosenbaum (1990; 1991a; 1991b) has published a number of articles outlining many dimensions of cultural care and health of Greek Canadian widows.

A review of qualitative research literature published in six major refereed nursing journals spanning the period of 1985 to 1990 uncovered no research studies that used the theory of cultural care as a theoretical framework (Reynolds, 1991). This finding reflects trends such as the general lack of identification of well organized nursing theoretical frameworks in qualitative research.

With the advent of the *Journal of Transcultural Nursing*, researchers using Leininger's theory have another vehicle for the publication of their work. This journal may promote an increase in the publication of research that uses her theory. Other sources that frequently include research using Leininger's theory are the proceedings of the National Care Conferences.

Future plans in the area of research are to continue to examine commonalities, patterns, and themes derived from the many researchers using the theory as a basis for building upon knowledge gained from research in the development of additional studies. After review of her work in 1988, Leininger concluded that:

> there are no universal or worldwide ethnocare concepts, but there are some recurrent care concepts such as (1) concern for, (2) attention to, (3) respect for, and (4) helping. More diversity in human care forms, meanings, processes and uses was found than universalities or similarities. (1988b, p. 29)

This finding remains true to the present day (Leininger, 1991a).

Leininger (1991a) provides a list of additional findings gleaned from studies using her theory. The results are the following: (a) care meanings and practices are difficult to ascertain because they are embedded in social structure, (b) cultural context and care values influence the expression and meaning of care, (c) to understand care meanings and uses often requires knowledge of the culture, (d) high technology nursing practices in Western cultures increases the distance between clients and nurses, (e) generic care is little understood and valued by nurses and other health providers, (f) key and general informants for the studies have expressed positive feelings about the research, and (g) clients believe that their ideas, beliefs, and lifeways must be understood by health providers before clients can be helped appropriately (Leininger, 1991a).

Implications of the research for further development of the theory also continues to be discussed. Leininger is focusing on these efforts by inviting selected researchers known to be using her theory to confer and examine research and theory issues. The results of a recent culture care theory invitational conference have yet to be published.

## Summary

The theory of culture care diversity and universality proposed by Madeleine Leininger is a useful guide for nursing practice, administration, education, and research. Two reasons why the theory is applicable to a wide range of nursing settings and situations are that the theory is broad in scope and it does not depend upon a definition of singular person as the object of the theory.

Leininger has clearly identified three major modes of nursing action for nursing practice: dimensions of the culture of nursing, described care facilitation, and resistance factors within the culture. Numerous undergraduate courses and curricula have been developed by Leininger and she has undertaken and directed a wide variety of research projects exploring aspects of culture care. Through these contributions, Leininger has demonstrated the applicability of her theory to the profession and discipline of nursing.

# References

American Nurses Association. (1986). *Cultural diversity in the nursing curriculum: A guide for implementation.* Kansas City, MO: Author.

Bohay, I. Z. (1991). Culture care meanings and experiences of pregnancy and childbirth of Ukrainians. In M. M. Leininger (Ed.), *Culture care diversity and universality: A theory of nursing.* New York: National League for Nursing.

Donaldson, S. K., & Crowley, D. M. (1978). The discipline of nursing. *Nursing Outlook, 26*(2), 113-120.

Fawcett, J. (1984). The metaparadigm to nursing: Present status and future refinements. *Image, 16*(34), 84-86.

Fawcett, J. (1989). *Analysis and evaluation of conceptual models of nursing.* Philadelphia: F. A. Davis.

Fitzpatrick, J., & Whall, A. (1989). *Conceptual models of nursing: Analysis and application.* Bowie, MD: Brady.

Gates, M. (1988). Caring behaviors experienced by couples during a hysterectomy. In M. M. Leininger (Ed.), *Care: Discovery and uses in clinical and community nursing.* Detroit, MI: Wayne State University Press.

Gates, M. (1991). Culture care theory for study of dying patients in hospital and hospice contexts. In M. M. Leininger (Ed.), *Culture care diversity and universality: A theory of nursing.* New York: National League for Nursing.

Gaut, D. (1981). Conceptual analysis of caring: Research method. In M. M. Leininger (Ed.), *Caring: An essential human need.* Thorofare, NJ: Charles B. Slack, 17-44.

Kloosterman, N. D. (1991). Cultural care: The missing link in severe sensory alteration. *Nursing Science Quarterly, 4*(3), 119-122.

Leininger, M. M. (1969). Ethnoscience: A promising research approach to improve nursing practice. *Image, 3*(1), 2-8.

Leininger, M. M. (1970). *Nursing and anthropology: Two worlds to blend.* New York: John Wiley.

Leininger, M. M. (1976). Towards conceptualization of transcultural health care systems: Concepts and a model. In M. M. Leininger (Ed.), *Transcultural health care issues and conditions*. Philadelphia, PA: F. A. Davis.

Leininger, M. M. (1977). Caring: The essence and central focus of nursing. The *phenomenon of caring: Part V*. Kansas City, MO: American Nurses Foundation.

Leininger, M. M. (1978). *Transcultural nursing: Concepts, theories and practices*. New York: John Wiley.

Leininger, M. M. (1980, October). Caring: A central focus of nursing and health care services. *Nursing and Health Care*, 135-176.

Leininger, M. M. (1981a). *Caring: An essential human need*. Thorofare, NJ: Charles B. Slack.

Leininger, M. M. (1981b). The phenomenon of caring: Importance, research questions and theoretical considerations. In M. M. Leininger (Ed.), *Caring: An essential human need*. Thorofare, NJ: Charles B. Slack.

Leininger, M. M. (1981c). Cross-cultural hypothetical functions of caring and nursing care. In M. M. Leininger (Ed.), *Caring: An essential human need*. Thorofare, NJ: Charles B. Slack.

Leininger, M. M. (1981d). Some philosophical, historical, taxonomic aspects of nursing and caring in American culture. In M. M. Leininger (Ed.), *Caring: An essential human need*. Thorofare, NJ: Charles B. Slack.

Leininger, M. M. (1984a). *Care: The essence of nursing and health*. Thorofare, NJ: Charles B. Slack.

Leininger, M. M. (1984b). Transcultural nursing: An overview. *Nursing Outlook*, 32(2), 72-73.

Leininger, M. M. (1984c). Southern rural black and white American lifeways with focus on care and health phenomena. In M. M. Leininger (Ed.), *Care: The essence of nursing and health*. Thorofare, NJ: Charles B. Slack.

Leininger, M. M. (1984d). Caring is nursing: Understanding the meaning, importance, and issues. In M. M. Leininger (Ed.), *Care: The essence of nursing and health*. Thorofare, NJ: Charles B. Slack.

Leininger, M. M. (1985a). Transcultural care diversity and universality: A theory of nursing. *Nursing and Health Care*, 6(4), 209-212.

Leininger, M. M. (1985b). Ethnography and ethnonursing: Models and modes of qualitative data analysis. In M. M. Leininger (Ed.), *Qualitative research methods in nursing* (pp. 33-32). Orlando, FL: Grune and Stratton.

Leininger, M. M. (1985c). Southern rural black and white American lifeways with focus on care and health phenomena. In M. M. Leininger (Ed.), *Qualitative research methods in nursing*. Orlando, FL: Grune and Stratton.

Leininger, M. M. (1986). Care facilitation and resistance factors in the culture of nursing. *Topics in Clinical Nursing*, 8(2), 1-12.

Leininger, M. M. (1988a). Leininger's theory of nursing: Cultural care diversity and universality. *Nursing Science Quarterly*, 1(4), 152-160.

Leininger, M. M. (1988b). History, issues, and trends in the discovery and uses of care in nursing. In M. M. Leininger (Ed.), *Care: Discovery and uses in clinical and community nursing*. Detroit: Wayne State University Press.

Leininger, M. M. (1988c). Cultural care theory and administration. In B. Henry, C. Arndt, M. Di Vincent, & A. Mariner-Tomey (Eds.), *Dimensions of nursing administration*. Boston, MA: Blackwell Scientific.

Leininger, M. M. (1988d). Leininger's theory of transcultural nursing: Culture care diversity and universality. *Nursing Science Quarterly, 2*(4), 11-20.

Leininger, M. M. (1989a). Transcultural nurse specialists and generalists: New practitioners in nursing. *Journal of Transcultural Nursing, 1*(1), 4-16.

Leininger, M. M. (1989b). Transcultural nursing: Quo vadis (where goeth the field). *Journal of Transcultural Nursing, 1*(l), 33-45.

Leininger, M. M. (1990a). Culture: the conspicuous missing link to understanding ethical and moral dimensions of human care. In M. M. Leininger (Ed.), *Ethical and moral dimensions of care*. Detroit, MI: Wayne State University Press.

Leininger, M. M. (1990b). Ethnomethods: The philosophic and epistemic bases to explicate transcultural nursing knowledge. *Journal of Transcultural Nursing, 1*(2), 40-51.

Leininger, M. M. (1991a). *Culture care diversity and universality: A theory of nursing.* New York: National League for Nursing.

Leininger, M. M. (1991b). Culture care of the Gadsup Akuna of the Eastern highlands of New Guinea. In M. M. Leininger (Ed.), *Culture care diversity and universality: A theory of nursing*. New York: National League for Nursing.

Leininger, M. M. (1993). Culture care theory: The comparative global theory to advance human care nursing knowledge and practice. In D. Gaut (Ed.), *A global agenda for caring* (pp. 3-18). New York: National League for Nursing.

Lincoln, Y., & Guba, E. (1985). *Qualitative research methods in nursing*. Orlando, FL: Grune and Stratton.

Luna, L. (1989). Transcultural nursing care of Arab Muslims. *Journal of Transcultural Nursing, 1*(1), 22-26.

Monsma, J. (1988) Children of battered women: Perceptions, actions, and nursing care implications. In M. M. Leininger (Ed.), *Care: Discovery and uses in clinical and community nursing*. Detroit, MI: Wayne State University Press.

Rosenbaum, J. (1988). Mental health care needs of Soviet-Jewish immigrants. In M. M. Leininger (Ed.), *Care: Discovery and uses in clinical and community nursing*. Detroit, MI: Wayne State University Press.

Rosenbaum, J. (1990). Cultural care of older Greek Canadian widows within Leininger's theory of culture care. *Journal of Transcultural Nursing, 2*(1), 37-47.

Rosenbaum, J. (1991a). Culture care theory and Greek Canadian widows. In M. M. Leininger (Ed.), *Culture care diversity and universality: A theory of nursing*. New York: National League for Nursing.

Rosenbaum, J. (1991b). Widowhood grief: A cultural perspective. *Canadian Journal of Nursing Research, 23*(2), 61-76.

Rosenbaum, J. (1991c). The health meanings and practices of older Greek Canadian widows. *Journal of Advanced Nursing, 16*, 1320-1327.

Reynolds, C. (1991). *The relationship between theory and qualitative research*. Unpublished manuscript.

Spangler, Z. (1991). Culture care of Philippine and Anglo-American nurses in a hospital context. In M. M. Leininger (Ed.), *Culture care diversity and universality: A theory of nursing.* New York: National League for Nursing.

Stasiak, D. B. (1991). Culture care theory with Mexican-Americans in an urban context. In M. M. Leininger (Ed.), *Culture care diversity and universality: A theory of nursing.* New York: National League for Nursing.

Steven, B. J. (1979). *Nursing theory: Analysis, application evaluation.* Boston: Little, Brown.

Tripp-Reimer, T., & Dougherty, M. C. (1985). Cross-cultural nursing research. In H. Werley & J. Fitzpatrick (Eds.), *Annual review of nursing research* (Vol. 3, pp. 77-104). New York: Springer.

Valentine, K. (1988). Advancing care and ethics in health management: An evaluation strategy. In M. M. Leininger (Ed.), *Care: Discovery of uses in clinical and community nursing* (pp. 151-168). Detroit, MI: Wayne State University Press.

Watson, J. (1985). *Nursing: Human science and human care: A theory for nursing.* Norwalk, CT: Appleton-Century-Crofts.

Wenger, A. F. Z., & Wenger, M. (1988). Community and family care patterns of the Old Order Amish. In M. M. Leininger (Ed.), *Care: Discovery and uses in clinical and community nursing.* Detroit, MI: Wayne State University Press.

Wenger, A. F. (1991). The culture care theory and the old order Amish. In M. M. Leininger (Ed.), *Culture care diversity and universality: A theory of nursing.* New York: National League for Nursing.

# About the Authors

**Cheryl L. Reynolds,** RN, PhD, served as a hospital corpsman in the U.S. Navy and the U.S. Naval Reserve and was awarded a special commendation with her honorable discharge. She received her Bachelor of Science in Nursing degree from Northern Michigan University in Marquette and her Master of Science degree from Arizona State University in Tempe. She has been a professor of nursing for the past 10 years at Northern Michigan University where she teaches both graduate and undergraduate students, has been instrumental in the development and delivery of the Adult Health Clinical Nurse Specialist program, and has received numerous awards and honors for her scholarship. Her area of special expertise is research and theory development related to health promotion phenomena. She was recently a doctoral student in nursing at Wayne State University, Detroit, where she studied the health promotion beliefs of the Ojibwe people.

**Madeleine M. Leininger,** RN, CTN, PhD, LHD, DS, PhD Nsc, FAAN, is Professor of Nursing and Anthropology, Wayne State University, Colleges of Nursing and Liberal Arts. She is an internationally known educator, author, theorist, administrator, researcher, consultant, and a frequently sought after public speaker. Her areas of expertise are transcultural nursing, comparative human care, qualitative research methods, cultural care theory, culture of nursing and health fields, anthropology, nursing, and the future of nursing. She established transcultural nursing as a formal field of study and practice, started the Transcultural Nursing Society (1974), and the International Association of Human Care (formerly the National Research Care Conference) (1978). She served as dean, professor of nursing, and director of the centers of nursing and health research at the University of Utah and Wayne State University.

Dr. Leininger is the author or editor of 25 books, 200 articles, chapters, and films. She has done extensive field research in Western and non-Western cultures. In the early 1960s, she was the first transcultural nurse to do an ethnographic and ethnonursing study with the Gadsup of the Eastern Highlands of New Guinea. Since then, she has done ethnonursing and ethnocare studies with a number of cultures ranging from Appalachia to Africa to the Philippines. She was an early leader in the development and use of qualitative research methods.